Medical Marijuana
*The History and Health Benefits
of Marijuana on Anxiety,
Cancer, Epilepsy, and More*

By Jake Allen

Table of Contents:

Introduction

Thank you for taking the time to check out *Medical Marijuana: The History and Health Benefits of Marijuana on Anxiety, Cancer, Epilepsy, and More.*

This book covers the topic of medical marijuana, and will teach you its history, laws, and practical uses.

At the completion of this book, you will have a good understanding of marijuana and be able to form an intelligent opinion on its use.

Chapter 1: What is Marijuana? What are the Health Benefits of Marijuana?

Marijuana is one of the oldest and most diversely useful psychoactive plants on Earth. Originally appearing among prehistoric societies throughout Euro-Asia and Africa, the oldest written record of marijuana dates to 440 BCE, when central Eurasian Scythians would take cannabis (another word for marijuana) steam baths. Greek historian Herodotus wrote, "The Scythians, as I said, take some of this hemp-seed and, creeping under the felt coverings, throw it upon the red-hot stones; immediate it smokes, and gives out such a vapor as no Grecian vapor-bath can exceed; the Scyths, delighted, shout for joy".

This is one of many records and depictions of marijuana and its many uses. What follows is a brief history and explanation of how this plant has impacted mankind throughout the world.

It is important to note that there are a variety of *types* of marijuana, which provide different uses unto themselves. The genus cannabis was first classified by Carl Linnaeus in the 17th century, whose naming system is still in use today. When describing the differences in the varieties, he noted that Indica strains seemed to have poorer fiber quality than Sativa (with Indica and Sativa being the two main species of marijuana). This classification also helped with the first step towards the industrialization and utilization of marijuana.

Throughout the 20th century, many botanists have argued and contested about the amount of marijuana strains that actually do exist as well as their function, though they all can agree that there are notable differences among the main varieties. In the 70s and 80s specifically, taxonomic classification of cannabis took on more weight, when North American laws prohibited specific strains (as some were more mind altering than others). These laws involved heated discussion from botanists on both sides of the fence, with both parties doing their best to discredit the other's knowledge.

In other parts of the world, however, great strides were being made to understand as well as create and categorize new types of cannabis, and determine medical uses for the leaf, stems and roots. Pharmacological uses specifically pushed scientists and corporations to further understand marijuana's medical application.

Once we entered the late 20th century, molecular analytical techniques were developed that helped classify and understand marijuana even more. Science has been able to dissect the actual RDNA of marijuana, primarily for plant breeding and forensic purposes.

At its current state, both here in the US (in legal states) and around the world, there couldn't be a better time to be in the marijuana industry as a scientist, entrepreneur, or a patient. Now, anyone can become involved in the scientific understanding of marijuana and the different ways you can produce, use, and consume the plant.

Outside of its vast medical uses, the other benefits of cannabis include utilizing the hemp fiber for oils, medicinal purposes, and as a recreational drug. Hemp describes the durable soft fiber from the plant stem, with some stems growing over six meters tall. The industrial hemp industry utilizes low THC (the psychoactive compound in marijuana) strains, to comply with the UN Narcotics Convention. At the opposite end of the spectrum, many high THC strains are grown to get the maximum psychoactive effects for both recreational and medicinal use.

Hemp can be turned into an almost limitless amount of products, ranging from paper, construction material for textiles, clothing, and cordage. The fibers of hemp are much stronger than traditional materials, and last much longer. Beyond construction materials, hemp can be turned into food, such as milk as well as biofuels.

Between 60 and 100 kilograms of cannabis are produced legally each year, with around 182.5 million cannabis users (around 4% of the population aged between 15-64).

Cannabis produces a few chemicals called cannabinoids, that affect people mentally and physically. Without getting too technical, cannabinoids, terpenoids, and other compounds within the flower are released through the combustion of the plant's fibers, which in turn interact with receptors within the human brain. It is important to note that the human brain is designed to receive the compounds released by marijuana, as this is notably different to how alcohol or other synthetic drugs affect the human body. We will get more into this in the later chapters on the medical uses of marijuana.

Currently, cannabis is illegal in most of the world, making it illegal to cultivate, possess or sell. Within the US (as well as other countries), some states have begun to make marijuana medicinally or recreationally legal, with a variety of positive outcomes.

Historically, there are vast ancient and religious uses of marijuana, spanning thousands of years and many cultures. The Yanghai Tombs, a large cemetery in the People's Republic of China, recently revealed the grave of a 2,700 year old shaman. Belonging to the Jushi culture, his body was discovered with a large leather basket and wooden bowl filled with almost 800 grams of marijuana, perfectly preserved. It even still contained active THC.

Other settlements dating from 2200-1700 BCE, possess ritual structures with rooms that contained all the tools necessary to make infusions from poppy, hemp, and ephedra. Even Hindu Vedas referred to cannabis in their Atharvaveda, being called the "food of the Gods". While Buddhists claim it could cloud your enlightenment, most practices regard cannabis as a powerful medical and spiritual tool, to be used properly and with discipline.

Over recent years, the outpouring of evidence pointing towards marijuana's positive health benefits has grown. Most notably, cannabis has been proven effective at aiding/treating epileptic seizures, glaucoma, lung issues, cancer, MS, HIV/AIDS, Hep-C, IBS, arthritis, Lupus, Crone's, Parkinson's, stroke, concussions, and trauma. Keep in mind that these are only a few of the physical health benefits of marijuana. Some of the mental benefits include the treatment or improvement of Alzheimer's, alcoholism, appetite, nightmares, creativity, PTSD, anxiety and depression, with more being discovered every day.

While the ways in which marijuana affect the human body to achieve these results vary, a comprehensive, 400-page analysis from the National Academies of Science, Engineering and Medicine, (nap.edu) was released this spring, and thoroughly covers the newest scientific research into the field, while also debunking some currently held beliefs about cannabis. In it, over 10,000 scientific studies were included, which came to over 100 conclusions regarding marijuana legislation, misinformation, and the overall agenda for and against cannabis. It also provides insights, filling missing gaps of information on the history of marijuana legalization and development.

Among the findings, the new report concludes that making marijuana a Schedule 1 drug creates administrative barriers for researchers to learn more about the plant that is saving lives. "It is often difficult for researchers to gain access to the quantity, quality, and type of cannabis product necessary to address specific research questions on the health effects of cannabis use", the article reads, concluded by a panel of experts led by Marie McCormick, from Harvard University.

The lack of support for research into medical marijuana is evident by the United States Federal Government's own cannabis program, which provides subpar plant material and insufficient funding. With the new administration here, it is unclear what will happen with the legalities of marijuana and its research.

The other main points of this article released by the NASEM were that cannabis and cannabinoids are effective at treating chronic pain, as well as pain from those suffering from other treatments, like chemotherapy. Cannabis is also not linked to the same types of cancers as those resulting from smoking, nor is it clear if it causes negative long term effects in adults.

While there is still much to be learned about how marijuana can affect the human body negatively over time, most of the studies from unbiased sources point to marijuana being one of the safest and most effective, natural medicines in existence.

Chapter 2: What are the Myths Surrounding Marijuana?

Besides the advent of the internet, misinformation and myths about marijuana truly began right after the Mexican revolution in the early 1900s. But before we get into the history of anti-marijuana propaganda and our public's current perception about the plant, let's discuss the different myths that surround marijuana.

Before much was known about the health effects of marijuana, many thought that it had similar physiological effects as smoking tobacco, or even drinking alcohol. In part, this is because one of the larger studies done on cannabis that was released a few years ago, which looked at the brains of 20 heavy cannabis users, and compared them to 20 non-smokers. The results displayed tissue differences in the brain, in areas related to cognitive and emotional processing. Major news outlets took the story and ran with it, claiming that marijuana "reorganizes the brain". While the author of this study explains that the results show only a slight correlation, the impression left from the media was not a positive one. This is one of the many ways our media has affected the true representation of marijuana.

Beyond the health-related myths that marijuana is carcinogenic or "depletes brain cells", there are a variety of societal myths and judgements falsely made against those who use cannabis medically or recreationally. Some of these myths include the notion that marijuana is addictive, even though the number of cannabis users who became dependent in a study from the 1990's was 9%, which is five percentage points below alcohol, and 15 percentage points below tobacco.

There is also the notion that marijuana users "look" a specific way, and possess characteristics to "pot-heads": lazy, hungry stoners who are a detriment to society, when in fact many highly successful people have admitted to using marijuana medicinally *and* recreationally as a way to naturally enhance and improve their mood, performance, and mind. Notable examples to this include Michael Phelps, Steve Jobs, Richard Branson, and many others. Companies and organizations who operate in medically legalized states, understand the importance and usefulness of cannabis to their employees, and allow smoke breaks for specific, "creativity-intensive" jobs.

These examples bust another myth about pot: That those who partake lack motivation. In fact, many of those who use cannabis for mental reasons, admit to it helping them face a considerably hard day, or relax after a particularly stressful evening.

As marijuana is still illegal throughout many states and many parts of the world, some rightfully believe that marijuana leads to troublemaking teens, as well as criminal activity. Sadly, these types of opinions are perpetuated largely by groups who would financially suffer if marijuana were to become legalized, but we'll get more into that in a moment. For now, the best explanation for the correlation between crime and marijuana, is the simple fact that marijuana *is* illegal, and that the laws, not the drug, were to blame. A Norwegian study specifically stated: "The study proposes that cannabis use in adolescence and young adulthood may be linked with subsequent involvement in criminal activity. However, the majority of this involvement seems to be related to different types of drug-specific crime. Thus, the association seems to rest on the fact that possession, use, and distribution of drugs such as cannabis is illegal. The study strengthens concerns about the laws related to the use, possession, and distribution of cannabis.

This myth, alongside of the myth that marijuana leads to harder drugs, is one of the main narratives that anti-marijuana groups use to fight and use legislation against cannabis. To understand why some groups would want marijuana to be illegal, we must first look at the years after the Mexican Revolution.

At this point in time in the United States, immigrants were heading into the country, bringing their cultures, customs, and language. This included the use of marijuana as a medicine.

While Americans were accustomed to cannabis (as it was available in different medicines and tinctures at that time), the way Mexicans spelled and spoke the word was foreign to them, spelling it marihuana instead of marijuana. When the media picked up on this, it began to create fear in the public about these unfamiliar citizens, and began wrongly spreading statements about disruptive Mexicans and their marijuana.

This demonization of the plant was actually just an extension of demonizing Mexicans. The US was trying to follow and control these new citizens, and it wasn't long until Paso, TX took a note out of San Francisco's playbook, which prohibited opium many decades before, as a way to take charge of immigrants from China. This was to have a reason to detain, examine, and deport immigrants from Mexico. And this reason became marijuana.

It wasn't long until this method became quite successful, eventually being adopted as a national strategy for managing some populations under control and watch.

In the 1930s, claims were being made about marijuana making men of color act violent, as well as solicit love acts from women who were white. This argument became the rallying cry of the Marijuana Tax Act of 1937, which definitively prohibited its use and sale. Years later this act was ruled unfair, and was reinstated with the Controlled Substances Act in the 1970s, which ranked substances based on their seriousness and potential for abuse. Ironically, cannabis was placed in the highest and most restricted category.

This was during Nixon's presidency, and he claimed that this placing of marijuana as a Schedule 1 drug was merely temporary, until he had time to revisit the case and make a final recommendation. This recommendation never came, and the Schafer Commission declared marijuana shouldn't exist in Schedule 1, and doubted its label as substance that is illicit. Nixon refused to acknowledge this claim and left marijuana as a Schedule 1 substance.

It wasn't until 1996 that California became the first state to accept the utilization of marijuana for medicinal reasons, which ended the 59-year outlawing of the plant as an illegal substance with no value for medicine. Before 1937, marijuana had a 5,000-year record as a therapeutic medicine across almost every culture. In context, making marijuana an illegal and hazardous drug was a mistake.

Regardless, those who opposed medical marijuana did so on the basis that there wasn't enough information to make a sound decision on its legality, without taking into account the nearly 5,000 years of known and documented work with cannabis throughout the world.

Since California's legalization, 23 other states including Washington, DC, have passed medical marijuana laws. At this point, a large portion of the public is wondering why it is still federally illegal and Schedule 1, especially considering the vast economic benefits that come from legalizing marijuana. Also, remember that myth that legalizing marijuana would increase crime? Colorado actually showed a reduction in crime, with a one billion dollar increase in revenue from taxing marijuana.

Beyond the natural development of how marijuana came to be here in the United States, there are other forces at work which attempt to keep marijuana illegal, including the tobacco and alcohol industry, different energy and textile industries, and the pharmacological industry. In fact, over 100,000 dollars were donated by an Arizona-based lobbying group which works for a pharmaceutical company that produces synthetic versions of marijuana. That's right: Instead of learning how to grow and produce marijuana to achieve its healing results, they lobbied against its legalization, in order to make profit on their synthetic version.

When hearing and seeing advertisements for or against marijuana, really try to understand why they are telling you their negative opinions on the topic. And just remember, many people are finding relief and healing from medicinal and recreational marijuana.

Chapter 3: Are There Any Risks to Marijuana?

It used to be incredibly difficult to find accurate information regarding the safety of using marijuana. In part this was because of lack of research. However, it is also because of how unregulated the collection of knowledge had been on the internet. Outside of visiting a library, which often wouldn't have the most current work and research on the topic, the only way to figure out the truth of cannabis was to try it yourself, trust your friends, and skeptically read any article you read on the internet.

Fortunately, things are a little different now. When searching for the risks of marijuana, the first links to come up are actually government sites that provide a surprisingly unbiased and fair look into the pros and cons of cannabis.

The first thing to note is there are both short term and long term effects to marijuana. In regards to short term effects, users may experience faulty body movement, the altered sense of time or other changed senses, difficulty problem solving, slight short term memory loss, and others.

While some users desire these effects, others prefer to get more of the medicinal effects of marijuana without the psychoactive effects. Fortunately, in areas where medicinal or recreational marijuana is legal, one is able to choose from a variety of strains and types, to suit their immediate needs. Whether you needed an uplifting, stimulating and creative high, or a very relaxed, warm and calm buzz, marijuana has truly become a specialized medicine for those who use it.

Concerning the long term effects; much is still unknown about marijuana. We do know that it affects brain development, and especially when used as a teenager or earlier, it can have known negative effects on the child's brain. It reduces one's ability to build connectors needed to continue learning and making sense of the world, which is vital when physiologically growing. Marijuana's effects on these parts of the brain may be long lasting or permanent, for the age range of child to late teenager.

As an example, a New Zealand study was conducted by researchers from Duke University showing that those who started habitual and heavy use of marijuana had a dropping average of eight IQ points between 13-38, with those points not showing back up later on in life. Some have argued that in this case, the aphorism, "ignorance is bliss", just might hold up.

Another important thing to note is the increase of THC within marijuana. Over the last few decades, as our scientific methods grow, and our pursuit for the purest product continues, we have been able to create higher levels of active cannabinoids within our medicinal products. This partially explains the rise of emergency room visits, as well as anecdotal stories through the news, where new patients or recreational users get "too high" for comfort, although their lives are never at risk, nor are they physically being harmed.

Other common health issues that could arise from habitual use of marijuana include breathing problems, increased heart rate, developmental disorders if using marijuana while pregnant, as well as a few, patient specific experiences, such as temporary hallucinations, temporary paranoia, and worsening symptoms of schizophrenia, for those already suffering from it.

For most, marijuana is the healthiest and safest option they have for treating whatever disease it's qualified to treat. As with all medicines, drugs, and herbal solutions, you should seek proper medical advice, and fully understand how pot interacts with different individuals. Part of this involves *how* you consume marijuana, the environment you put yourself in, and the things you do while on the substance. Read on to learn more about the different ways to use and benefit from marijuana.

Chapter 4: Different Ways to Consume Marijuana

While the ways you can consume marijuana have stayed the same, the ways you can process the plant have grown dramatically. In part, this is because of new technological advancements, as well as the need for marijuana to meet state and federal laws. Before we dive into the different processes and end products of marijuana, let's briefly discuss the different ways you can consume it.

Traditionally, marijuana has been smoked, or cooked and orally consumed via different recipes. The most straightforward way to smoke marijuana is by taking the dry leaf, removing the stems, breaking the cured leaf apart, and putting it into a smoking pipe or wrapping it in rolling papers. When it comes to ingesting marijuana, many have made the mistake of eating the raw leaf itself, or steeping it in tea for a time before drinking it. The problem with this, is that the cannabis is not yet activated. What this means, is that in order for marijuana to become active (or respond to the human body), it must first be brought to a temperature where the compounds are accelerated and become bioavailable.

So, before turning your marijuana leaf into butter, oil, or a tea, you must first bring you marijuana to its decarboxylation point. Different temperatures will activate, burn, or preserve different compounds in the cannabis, and the rabbit hole can go quite deep when it comes to creating your own edibles.

Outside of smoking or ingesting marijuana, you can also apply it topically, through the use of a cream or oil. At one point, there was a huge scientific hurdle and challenge between turning raw leaf into processed, useable goods, but since its legalization in California, many tech companies and investors have spent considerable money making its access and use very straightforward.

This research has yielded a variety of new marijuana products, which go by an almost endless stream of names: Errl, shatter, wax, butter, churn, and crumble. These are words to describe extracts. Extracts are exactly what the name implies - highly concentrated versions of marijuana.

Growers and dispensaries achieve this type of product by using machines called extractors, as well as gases or liquids such as CO_2 and butane, to pull the active compounds of marijuana out of the plant. This creates different consistencies based on when you take it out of the extractor, and at what temperature you extract the marijuana at.

The benefits to this product are numerous, from streamlining the creation of edibles, to making marijuana completely mobile, discrete (and respectful of other people's spaces), and less damaging on the body, as you are taking less smoke in regularly over time. It is also considerably more expensive than traditional leaf, but this is in part due to the process it has to go through and the type of equipment used in its processing. It's reported that between 1/7th and 1/10th of the marijuana used in extraction is salvaged and can be used for consumption. Talk about a costly process!

Chapter 5: Medicinal Marijuana and State/Federal Laws

In the last twenty-some odd years, the term medical marijuana has become an ecosystem unto itself. In this chapter we'll discuss what medical marijuana means, as well as the different state and federal laws regarding the regulation, sale, and consumption of marijuana.

In its most basic form, medical marijuana means: "Marijuana that has been recommended by a doctor in the treatment of a medical condition". In 1966, when California voters passed Prop 215, the government needed to determine what using medical marijuana meant for the patient, and needed to create laws from scratch to protect the rights of those seeking cannabis for medicinal reasons.

The National Conference of State Legislature uses a criterion similar to the one California created, and uses this criteria to determine if new programs introduced are comprehensive or not.

These rules and laws allow:
1. Protection from criminal punishment for using marijuana for a medical reason
2. Access to marijuana through home gardens, dispensaries or some other system that is likely to be in place

3. It allows a variety of strains, including those more than "low THC"

4. It allows either vaporization or smoking of some kinds of marijuana compounds, plant extract or material

In acknowledgment to California's Prop 215, the Institute of Medicine issues a report that sought to find the therapeutic uses for marijuana. The report suggested that, "scientific data indicate potential therapeutic value of cannabinoid drugs, primarily THC, for pain relief, control of nausea and vomiting, and appetite stimulation; smoked marijuana, however, is a crude THC delivery system that also provides harmful substances. The psychological effects of cannabinoids, such as anxiety reduction, sedation, and euphoria can influence their potential therapeutic value. Those effects are potentially undesirable for certain patients and situations and beneficial for others. In addition, psychological effects can complicate the interpretation of other aspects of the drug's effect". In short, this study confirmed why California was moving towards legalization in the first place.

While states provide specific rights to those who use medical marijuana, their perspective is very different than the federal government. At the federal level, marijuana remains classified as a schedule 1 substance, where it is suggested that marijuana possesses a high abuse potential. However, in October 2009, the Obama administration delivered a memo to federal prosecutors telling them not to punish people who distribute marijuana for medicinal purposes in accordance with state law. The US Department of Justice, in August 2013, made a revision to their medical marijuana policy with their new statement reading that while marijuana still is federally against the law, the USDOJ expects states like Washington and Colorado to form powerful, state-based enforcement endeavors, and that they will defer the right to object to their laws for legalization at this time.

While many states have made marijuana medicinally legal, multiple states have overturned the ruling since, including Arizona, and the District of Columbia. In 1996, Arizona voters initially passed a ballot initiative. Unfortunately, this initiative said that doctors would be permitted to write a "prescription" for marijuana. As marijuana is a substance from Schedule 1, federal law forbids providing a prescription, which made the initiative false.

To work around this, states that have medical marijuana laws in place have a type of patient registry, which provides security against arrest for possession (up to a certain point), for medical reasons.

With the introduction of medicinal marijuana legislation, there have been a host of common policy questions concerning how to manage its recommendations, its dispensing, and the registering of patients who are approved. Some states do not have a regulation on dispensary, and because of this, they could experience a financial boom in business, until more strict regulations are made. Those who grow marijuana and provide it to patients are normally called "caregivers". Caregivers are usually restricted in the amount of marijuana they are able to grow. Below is a description of every states' medical marijuana laws, including if the state provides a patient registry, allows dispensaries, and permits retail sales. Unless otherwise noted, if there is no mention of retail sales for that specific state, the state does not allow it.

Alaska made medical marijuana legal in 1998, and was one of the first states to introduce the patient registry. While the state does not currently allow for dispensaries, it is in the process of creating its retail operation.

Arizona became medically legal in 2010, provides a patient registry, allows for dispensaries and allows patients from other states to purchase marijuana.

California was legalized originally by Prop 215, which was ratified to SB420 in 2003. This allows for dispensaries and provides a patient registry, and also allows retail sales (through Prop 64)

Colorado became medically legal in 2000, provides patients with a registry and a dispensary, though it does not allow patients from other states to purchase medical marijuana.

Connecticut was legalized in 2012, and does provide a patient registry, with permits for dispensaries. Connecticut does not recognize patients from other states.

Delaware has had medical marijuana since 2011, and afford patients a registry and the ability to sell through dispensaries, though it does not allow interstate purchasing.

The District of Columbia passed its medical marijuana initiative in 2010, and it affords patients a registry, dispensaries, and allows patients from other states to purchase marijuana in DC.

Florida recently passed Amendment 2 in 2016, though all details are still pending.

Guam currently provides medical marijuana, a registry, and dispensaries, and has since 2015.

Hawaii passed SB 862 in 2000, which provides a patient registry, but does not allow dispensaries.

Illinois has HB 1 (passed in 2013), and it includes a patient registry and dispensaries, but does not allow patients from other states to purchase marijuana.

Maines most recent bill was LD 1296, passed in 2011. This bill does permit a patient registry, as well as dispensaries, and also allows for retail sales, and interstate purchasing (just not through dispensaries).

Maryland's current bill is HB 881, and it allows for a patient registry, dispensaries, but no interstate purchasing.

Massachusetts made medical marijuana legal in 2013, and provides everything except interstate purchasing.

Michigan's medical marijuana bill was passed in 2008, and while it does provide a patient registry, it does not provide dispensaries, and only recognizes interstate purchases for legal protection of possession, and not for dispensary purchases.

Minnesota's initiative, SF 2471, has a patient registry, but very limited amount of purchasable marijuana through their dispensaries.

Montana made medical marijuana legal in 2016, and provides a patient registry, with new details coming about dispensaries and interstate purchases.

Nevada's Question 9, made legal in 2000, does allows a patient registry, but doesn't allow dispensaries. Nevada does however, provide retail sales and allows for interstate purchases.

New Hampshire's HB 573 permits interstate purchasing with a note from their home state, and also includes a patient registry and dispensaries.

New Jersey passed SB 119 in 2009, and affords patients a registry, dispensaries, but no interstate purchasing.

New Mexico's SB 523 was passed in 2007, and give patients a registry, access to dispensaries, but no interstate purchasing.

New York passed their initiative in 2014, and provides a registry, but strict laws regarding the consumption of THC, including ingested doses not containing more than 10mg of THC, and that the product may not be smoke (so only ingested).

North Dakota's Measure 5 was instated in 2016, with all details of their bill still pending.

Ohio's newest bill allowing medical marijuana was signed in 2016, but the details are not currently available and it is not in effect yet.

Oregon's Medical Marijuana act of 1998 was one of the first steps towards legalization of medical marijuana, and permits a patient registry, but no dispensaries (although you can purchase marijuana for recreational use).

Pennsylvania's medical marijuana initiative was signed by the governor in 2016, but it is not yet operational. It does allow for a patient registry and dispensaries.

Puerto Rico passed the Public Health Department Regulation 155 in 2016, but no details of the law is available, and it is not yet operational.

Rhode Island's SB 185 permits a patient registry, a dispensary, and it recognizes interstate purchases.

Vermont passed SB 17 in 2011, and provides dispensaries, a patient registry, but not interstate purchases.

Washington's initiative SB 5073 does not provide a patient registry, but it does allow for permits, and recreational sales. It is important to note Washington does not allow interstate purchases.

West Virginia's initiative SB 386 is still waiting for the signature of the governor, but would allow for a patient registry, a dispensary, but you cannot combust or smoke the leaf (it must be vaporized or ingested).

The details of each states laws can and do change regularly, and it's a good idea to check up on the most current version of each states laws. In the next chapter, we'll discuss the variety of ailments marijuana helps treat, and dive into the history and science behind this medicinal plant.

Chapter 6: What Can Marijuana Treat?

For over 5,000 years, marijuana has had a history of treating a variety of health-related issues. In fact, very few plants have as extensive of a history as a miracle herb like marijuana; used by shamans, healers, teachers, students, philosophers, and your average everyman, for millennium. Starting from 2900 BCE, we are going to go through history and discuss the different ways marijuana has been used in positive, life healing ways.

As far back as 3000 BCE, Chinese Emperors have been recorded referencing marijuana as a popular medicine, possessing both yin and yang in its properties. It wasn't until 2700 BCE, however, that Chinese Emperor Shen Nung was believed to have discovered the healing wonders of medicine. Shen Nung was considered the father of Chinese medicine, and also discovered ginseng and ephedra.

Around 1500 BCE, the earliest written reference to medical marijuana was found within the Chinese Pharmacopeia, the Rh-Ya. In 1450, Exodus' book refers to cannabis-made holy anointing oil. This was explained in the Exodus Hebrew version (30:22-23), and consisted of kaneh bosem, more than six pounds of the substance, which is described by respected anthropologists, researchers, etymologists, and botanists, as marijuana.

On the other side of the world, around 1212 BCE, Egyptians used cannabis for enemas, glaucoma, inflammation, and even the cooling of the uterus. The pollen of cannabis was discovered on the mummy of Ramesses the second, who expired in 1213 BCE.

At 1000 BCE, Bhang, a beverage made of milk and cannabis, was used an anesthetic used in India, and it was also used as an anti-phlegmatic. Then, in 700 BCE, the Middle East's use of marijuana was catalogued in the *Venidad*. The *Venidad* is one of the parts of the *Zend-Avesta*, the religious book of the ancient Persians, which was written near the seventh century BCE, supposedly by Zoroaster (or Zarathustra), who is said to be the creator of Zoroastrianism. He listed bhang (marijuana) as one of the most important of 10,000 medicinal plants.

Around 600 BCE, *Indian Medicine Treatise* cited the use of cannabis as leprosy's cure. Used as a medical application, people believe it could make the mind work more quickly, make life last longer, reduce high fevers, induce sleep, and cure dysentery. *The Ayurvedic System* and Treatise of *Sushruta Samhita*, written in 600 BCE, cited cannabis as a cure for leprosy and as an anti-phlegmatic.

The medical type of cannabis was also used in ancient Greece as a treatment for inflammation, edema, and earache. Right before the transition of BCE to AD, ancient Chinese writing advocates marijuana for over 100 ailments, which included absentmindedness, rheumatism, gout, and malaria. At the same time, Jesus apparently used oil for anointing composed of cannabis. This discovery, found in the New Testament bible, divined that Jesus anointed his 12 disciples (or followers) with a very strong entheogenic (psychoactive substance), and then made the followers do the exact same thing, close to the year 30 AD.

In ancient Rome, medical text cited cannabis as a treatment to earaches as well as a sexual suppressant. Pedanius Dioscorides was a Roman army doctor and a Greek physician who traveled widely on various campaigns with the Roman empire. He also reviewed and studied many varieties of plants, and put his findings within a text he called *De Materia Medica (On Medical Matters).* It was printed around 70 AD, and became the go-to text for medical knowledge over the next 1500 years. It concluded that cannabis, the male *and* female plant, were useful in making rope, and producing a juice to treat earache.

A bit later (80AD), a Roman nobleman named Pliny, wrote that cannabis roots, when boiled down, relieve gout, joints that are cramped, and help alleviate terrible pain. Chinese surgeon Hua T'o also referenced cannabis, as an effective anesthetic and also a compelling wine.

Fast-forward 600 years, and cannabis can be found being used as medicine in the Arabic world. At the same time, others in the same world where calling marijuana "lethal poison", although the claim was baseless and came from one Arab physician named Ibn Wahshiyah.

In 1500, marijuana was being used to reduce sexuality by Moslem doctors. Alongside of this, hemp was being used during the middle ages, with William Turner (a naturalist) popularizing it in the *New Herbal*, his own book, published in 1538.

50 years later, a text called the *Bencao Gangmu Materia Medica*, written by Li SHizhen, chronicles the utilization of marijuana to help aid a variety of human maladies, like parasites, vomiting, and hemorrhage. It continues to be used to this day for diarrhea, dysentery, and to stimulate the appetite.

Around the mid 1600's, some historians believe that William Shakespeare might have smoked marijuana. In the Journal of Science from South Africa, Thackeray reported identification of the chemical analyses of the residue of plants in tobacco popes, dating back to the early 17th century. The pipes had been procured on loan through Shakespeare's Birthplace Trust. Results from this study indicated that marijuana was in eight of the 24 samples, and in at least one sample, there was evidence of Peruvian cocaine!

Between 1611 to 1762, it is believed the Jamestown Settlers brought marijuana to North America. Virginia actually awarded many riches for hemp culturing and manufacturing, and also punished various people who refused to grow it.

Meanwhile, in England, Robert Burton, an Oxford scholar and English Clergyman, suggested that cannabis is a useful cure for the symptoms of depression. This can be found in his popular book titled *The Anatomy of Melancholy*. Herbalist Nicholas Culpepper also wrote about his positive experiences with marijuana as a medicine, writing that the extract in hemp, "allayed inflammations in the head ... eases the pains of the gout ... knots in the joints, [and] the pains of the sinews and hips". Culpeper's configuration probably had a small amount of psychoactivity as native cannabis cultivated in latitudes of the north has relatively low tetrahydrocannabinol (THC) matter."

Believe it or not, George Washington himself grew marijuana: According to his diary entries, he cultivated the hemp plant at his plantation of Mount Vernon, for around 30 years. As stated in the ledgers he kept, it appears that he had a specific fascination in the medical use of marijuana, and grew THC specific strains. Thomas Jefferson, a co-patriot, grew hemp at Monticello. This was noted in his own farming diaries, although there was no note as to whether or not he was a habitual smoker of the leaf, or of any type of leaf, for that matter. In Jefferson's farm book, he speaks on dividing female and male hemp plants, and some argue this is evidence for his desire to get strains that are consumable and potent.

Right before the turn of the 17th century, Napoleon's forces brought cannabis from Egypt to France. A scientific expedition team was researching the drug for its sedating and pain-relieving effects, while it was becoming more prominent in our western culture.

It wasn't long after, in 1840, that medical marijuana came to the UK through William O'Shaughnessy. It is reported that Queen Victoria used the plant for menstrual cramps. William was an army surgeon who served in the Indian war. He prescribed the medicine for a variety of ailments, including rheumatism, convulsions, tetanus, rabies, epilepsy, and also to promote uterine contractions in childbirth.

Marijuana was becoming more mainstream as a medicine used in the western part of the world around the 19th century. Jacques-Joseph Moreau, a French doctor, discovered that marijuana alleviated the pain caused by headaches, increased people's appetites, and caused people to become sleepy. Then, in the 1850s, marijuana was added to the US Pharmacopeia, which was an official standard-settings authoritative book that listed all prescriptions and over-the-counter drugs. It too listed cannabis as medicine for various ailments, including typhus, tetanus, dysentery, cholera, rabies, alcoholism, anthrax, convulsive disorders, addiction to opiates, leprosy, gout, insanity, incontinence, tonsillitis, extreme menstrual bleeding, neuralgia, and more. At this time, patents on marijuana tinctures were being sold.

In the 1800's and 1900's, marijuana wasn't the only thing being introduced to the west. Opium was also becoming increasingly popular, with opiate withdrawal becoming a very real thing for its users. An article was released in 1889 that outlined how to use marijuana for dealing with opium withdrawal. This article, written by Dr. E.A.Birch in *The Lancet* (one of the nation's most trusted medical texts), instructed users to smoke or drink the concoction for reduction of opiate and chloral hydrate withdrawal.

Right at the turn of the 20th century, the Indian Hemp Commission mentioned marijuana as a medical tool, being an increaser of energy, a powerful analgesic, an ecbolic, a hemostat, and an anti-diuretic. It's also believed to be an aid in helping treat cholera, gonorrhea, hay fever, dysentery, impotence, urinary incontinence, diabetes, swelling, granulation of open sores, and chronic ulcers. Other benefits include the prevention of insomnia, abatement of hunger, and as a treatment to help with the concentration of attention.

In South Asia, cannabis was used for bronchitis, asthma, and loss of appetite throughout the 1900s. Alongside of this, the Pure Food and Drugs Act requires the labeling of all medicine, in addition to cannabis. President Roosevelt signed this act into existence (known as the Wiley act). This stated, "an Act for preventing the manufacture, sale, or transportation of adulterated or misbranded or poisonous or deleterious foods, drugs, medicines, and liquors, and for regulating traffic therein, and for other purposes. That for the purposes of this Act an article shall also be deemed to be misbranded... if the package fail to bear a statement on the label of the quantity or proportion of any alcohol, morphine, opium, cocaine, heroin, alpha or beta eucaine, chloroform, cannabis Indica, chloral hydrate, or acetanilide, or any derivative or preparation of any such substances contained therein.".

Then, in 1911, Massachusetts became the first state to outlaw cannabis. This took place around the same time as alcohol prohibition in America, though it was banned for different reasons. President Wilson at the time signed the Harrison Act in 1913, which introduced three bills to try to fix the problem with opium use. Though this Act wasn't about marijuana, it did set the precedent for the government to regulate and register medicines (with cannabis eventually being one of them).

Soon after Massachusetts, 10 other states passed marijuana prohibition laws. The states that passed these laws were: Wyoming, Utah, Texas, Nevada, Iowa, Oregon, Washington, Arkansas, Nebraska, and New York. This all took place between 1915 and 1927.

Although many states moved to make marijuana illegal, the US pharmaceutical farm grows 60,000 pounds of marijuana annually for many years and up until WWI. The US became self-sufficient in its cannabis dependence in 1913, to be used for different industrial and medicinal purposes. Then, on February 19th, 1925, the League of Nations signed a multilateral treaty limiting cannabis to be used for medicinal and scientific purposes.

With new regulations around marijuana, American Pharmaceutical companies see a rise in demand for the medicinal qualities of cannabis. As such, they ramp up their product of marijuana extracts, which mainly acted as an analgesic, an antispasmodic, and a sedative. Marijuana cigarettes were sold for the treatment of asthma.

While a variety of new legislation is introduced over the remainder of the 1900s, meant to restrict and control the use of marijuana, there is also a growing body of scientific evidence uncovering new uses for medical marijuana. One of the first great achievements was the identification of synthesis of THC, which allowed researchers to pinpoint and study the active compounds in marijuana, and create specialized medicines based on the amount of these compounds. In fact, the University of Mississippi became the first official grower for the Federal Government, which was used to find different uses and medical solutions from medical cannabis.

To date, cannabis has treated and continues to treat over 150 different types of physical and mental issues, ailments, diseases, and challenges. In the coming chapters, we will discuss a few of the most challenging physical and mental illnesses of our times, and how marijuana is helping treat them.

Chapter 7: Psychological Benefits of Medical Marijuana

Only in the last twenty years has science been able to study and analyze the effects of marijuana on a human being's psychology. Thanks to the advent of neuroscience, we can see exactly how neural pathways interact with different medicines, and observe improvements or degradation of nerves and cells.

One of the most common uses of marijuana has been for pain management. Chronic pain, leading to a reduced quality of life, is one of the leading causes of suffering. Those who experience chronic pain understand how difficult it is to make it through a day.

Fortunately, with cannabis, the active compounds in the plant actually provide neuropathic pain reduction by affecting the frontal limbic cannabinoid receptors, as well as reducing the activity in the amygdale and primary sensorimotor regions, marijuana has provided therapy for many suffering from chronic pain. More research is being done daily to understand how marijuana specifically alleviate pains, with some scientists suggesting that it provides "distractive therapy", where the patient is able to focus on other things in their life instead of the suffering that is in front of them. This is different from a drug like opium, which attaches to the feel-good centers of the brain and blocks out the negative feelings.

Another psychological benefit of marijuana is its ability to function as an antidepressant. While scientists still don't know how cannabis acts as a mood booster, we do observe the release of dopamine and anandamide, which produces a relaxing effect. More research needs to be done concerning the long-term efficacy of using marijuana as an antidepressant, but short-term use does seem to be effective for many patients.

When it comes to aggression and hostility, marijuana is one of the ultimate counter balances. A natural way to control mood without antidepressants, marijuana has been shown to reduce aggression even in those who were exposed to a frustration stimulus.

Being able to sleep is a crucial part of having a healthy psychology. Many doctors believe sleep and dreaming are the times when our brain can organize and make sense of our memories and experiences. Anyone who suffers from insomnia understands how difficult it is to maintain a positive mood and mindset when you are unable to sleep.

Fortunately, marijuana has been shown to be an incredibly useful sleep aid. Not only that, but many patients testify that cannabis helps with their anxiety, PTSD, stress, and gives them the ability to relax. At the other end of the spectrum, some users do experience higher levels of anxiety and an inability to relax when using marijuana, but doctors who advise patients on medical marijuana say that this is because of improper dosing or choosing the incorrect strain for the type of issue the patient is having. Many strains are made without psychoactive compounds, and even some states in the US have legalized CBD-only strains, which contain zero THC and help users experiencing intense pain from cancer, western treatments, and other illnesses or pain-inducing procedures.

Other users of marijuana report an increase in creativity and energy, and there have even been reports of cannabis helping reduce patients' OCD and general obsessions. By allowing the brain to calm down and focus on the thing that is in front of them, marijuana patients often prefer the natural solution of marijuana to alternative medicines such as MAOI's and SSRI's, as their side effects are much more mild.

Some patients have reported development of their spiritual selves, noticing a lack of resentment and an observation of growth and compassion towards others and the world. While scientists are still trying to discover exactly what compounds in marijuana affect patient's brains in this way, it is important to remember that marijuana has been taking care of these types of needs for thousands of years, long before there were laboratories to take apart the structure of marijuana. Throughout history our ancestors have used marijuana to gain access into different parts of their personality and moods, and marijuana has helped create some of the most beautiful works of art and ideas.

Chapter 8: Medicinal Marijuana and Epilepsy

Besides psychological benefits, the scientific community has begun to discover that marijuana might possess extensive benefits to patients suffering from epilepsy. In fact, new studies are launching all over the world, trying to identify exactly what compounds are initiating the relief found in medical marijuana. The reason there is still any uncertainty about marijuana's efficacy towards the treatment of seizures is due to the lack of evidence and access to the plants and patients needed to perform these studies.

The amount of clinical studies performed has been small. One of them found that cannabis possesses a compound called cannabidiol (CBD), a non-psychoactive element, which could be responsible for the relief. Research of drugs derived from cannabidiol is currently being performed, and those drugs are prescribed to patients suffering from epilepsy.

Recently, double-blind placebo controlled studies were done on illnesses such as the Lennox-Gastaut syndrome and the Dravet syndrome. The parameters of these studies were that people who received the CBD drug range from 2-26 years old, and they all had seizures that did not respond to currently available treatments. What these studies found were that seizures decreased by an average of 54% while using the CBD-synthesized drug.

Another study, performed in Israel, used a product that had 20 parts of CBD to 1 part THC on children up to 18 years of age. A significant number of people reported seizure reduction, with 7% stating seizure worsening.

While this is great news for those who suffer from epilepsy, there still needs to be more research in the area. Many believe since CBD is an oil, it is less harmful than other drugs one can be prescribed, when in reality, CBD is broken down in your liver just like any other type of drug.

Fortunately, most of the side effects of CBD are much less harmful than other prescription medicines for seizures. These side effects include sleepiness, diarrhea, fatigue, and decreased appetite.

It is important to note that these are side effects from synthesized versions of CBD and not marijuana in its pure form. This is important, in part, because we do not know if the same challenges occur from taking the natural version of the medicine. Also, there have been signs of drug-to-drug interactions with the synthesized CBD medicine. It appears that people who had increases in their liver enzymes were also on valproic acid, which is an anti-seizure medication. What this means is that CBD may interact with VPA when it is broken down, increasing your risk for liver issues. Also, when clobazam is broken down, its major part appears to interact with CBD and cause tiredness.

Beyond the new science surrounding seizures and medicinal marijuana, it is important to note that stories of cannabis's ability to alleviate seizures has been around for about 150 years. Its legalization has allowed us the ability to research cannabis and its medicinal properties.

Chapter 9: Medicinal Marijuana and Cancer

As we said in the previous chapter, the legalization of marijuana has been one of the best things to happen to the research of its medical properties in the last 100 years. Before we get into if and how marijuana is effective in the treatment of cancer, it's important to understand the other current treatments that exist.

To begin with, surgery has been one of the main ways of taking out cancer. By removing bulk tumors, doctors are able to alleviate pain and pressure. Surgeons usually also remove healthy tissue and lymph nodes for research as well.

Radiation is one of the other more popular solutions, sending high doses into your body week after week, hoping to slow or kill the tumors completely. Unfortunately, this can take months, while also destroying healthy tissue as well.

Chemotherapy is similar to radiation, in that they hurt both good and bad cells. Chemotherapy does this by administering chemicals into the blood stream.

Immunotherapy is a type of biological therapy that makes use of organisms to stimulate the immune system, and this often gives patients symptoms similar to the flu.

Hormones are usually given via injection, orally, or while a person is undergoing surgery. This also acts to halt or slow down the production of cancerous cells, and helps lower and prevent symptoms of cancer from appearing. It is often utilized with different forms of treatment, and the side effects usually include diarrhea, fatigue, and nausea (with the chance to weaken bones and chance women's menstrual cycles).

Finally, heat (which can also be referred to as local hyperthermia) can kill minuscule parts of cells, while whole body and regional hyperthermia are used in combination with various treatments in order to make them perform more efficiently. It can be created externally, or internally, depending on the location of the cancer.

So how does cannabis fit in with all of this? Cannabis contains around 90 types of cannabinoids, which as we discussed, is the active chemical that creates different effects throughout the body (with some of these being psychoactive). The impact that these cannabinoids has on cancer and treating cancer symptoms is so powerful, that these cannabinoids are synthesized for legal prescription use. Two synthetic pill forms of THC, named Dronabinol and Nabilone, are FDA-approved, and are also used to treat vomiting and nausea that results from chemo.

So what are the cannabinoids that benefit people suffering from cancer, and what do these compounds actually do? Well, the compounds are CBC, CBD, CBDa, CBG, THC, and THCa, and they mainly help with inflammation, anxiety, and reduce pain. Other effects of these cannabinoids include the blocking of bad growth of cells, and blocking the production of blood vessels that fund tumors, as well as wrestling viruses and relieving spasm.

The National Cancer Institute also acknowledges that smoking marijuana helps with improved mood and sense of well-being in cancer patients, with studies suggesting that symptom management can take place by preventing vomiting, improving hunger, easing pain symptoms, and advancing sleep.

Some noteworthy studies include a study from 1996, which found the defensive effects of cannabinoids on the production of various tumor forms. They were viewed causing the death of cells, suggesting that cannabinoids could decimate cancer cells while keeping normal ones safe. Also, in 2003, a serious of studies on brain tumors proved that CBD may make chemotherapy a more useful treatment, and raise the death of cancer cells without hurting normal cells.

This complemented a study on mice in 2004, which revealed that cannabinoids protected against colon inflammation, which reduced the risk of colon cancer and potentially aided in its treatment. The American Association for Cancer Research demonstrated in the beginning of 2011 that CBD destroys cells linked to cancer of the breast, while not having any effect on usual breast cells. CBD also lowered the growth, spread, and number of tumors in mice.

In 2011, the National Institute of Health released a study called *Cell Death and Differentiation* that demonstrated JWH-015 (a receptor of a cannabinoid) and THC decrease the strength of cancerous cells in the liver. In addition, these cannabinoids were shown to decrease the production of tumors and the amount of fluid in the abdomen. These are huge discoveries because they could be useful in the creation of therapies that regulate liver cancer.

Further, a February 2015 study discovered that the risk of bladder cancer is 45% lower in cannabis patients. As claimed by the National Cancer Institute, studies show efficacy in cannabinoids and lung cancer. These cannabinoid receptors on the brain, spinal cord, and nerve endings within the body, now suggest marijuana might play a bigger role in our bodies' ecosystem and healing processes.

From the American Cancer Society's website on their stance towards marijuana and cancer patients: "The American Cancer Society supports the need for more scientific research on cannabinoids for cancer patients, and recognizes the need for better and more effective therapies that can overcome the often-debilitating side effects of cancer and its treatment. The Society also believes that the classification of marijuana as a Schedule 1 controlled substance by the US Drug Enforcement Administration imposes numerous conditions on researchers and deters scientific study of cannabinoids. Federal officials should examine options consistent with federal law for enabling more scientific study on marijuana.

Medical decisions about pain and symptom management should be made between the patient and his or her doctor, balancing evidence of benefit and harm to the patient, the patient's preferences and values, and any laws and regulations that may apply.

The American Cancer Society Cancer Action Network (ACS CAN), the Society's advocacy affiliate, has not taken a position on legalization of marijuana for medical purposes because of the need for more scientific research on marijuana's potential benefits and harms. However, ACS CAN oppose the smoking or vaping of marijuana and other cannabinoids in public places because the carcinogens in marijuana smoke pose numerous health hazards to the patient and others in the patient's presence."

With medical marijuana gaining traction and support from a variety of doctors, establishments, governments, and countries, we live in a time where our options for treating our diseases are broad. The most current forms of treatment for cancer with marijuana includes consuming oral CBD to treat solid tumors, treating repeating glioblastoma multiforms with a THC/CBD mouth spray, and treating graft-versus-host disease with CBD in victims who have had transplants dealing with stem cells.

Beyond the treatment of cancers symptoms, there is also the question of if marijuana can cure cancer. Considering that just under 40% of Americans will be diagnosed with cancer at some point in their lives, chances are you or someone you know will be confronted with it.

Perhaps not surprisingly, oncologists recommend marijuana as part of a treatment program for patients suffering from cancer more than any other medical professional. And even though the positive effects of marijuana have been recorded for 5,000 years, the US government still classifies it as a drug belonging to Schedule 1 class, with "a huge potential for abuse and no known medical use". Because of this, there's a good chance our progress and search to understand if pot is a cure for cancer will continue to be stifled and held up.

The other challenge is understanding what the word "cure" means. Usually, it means a patient has survived for 5 years without any symptoms or evidence of their cancer. For incurable diseases, however, this instead means an increase in one's pain management, and the quality of life that a patient experiences. Dr. Abrams, a leading supporter of marijuana and top oncologist, posits that around 33% of his patients have sought out marijuana as part of their treatment package, on their own accord, before it started becoming legal in the United States.

If this is true, then around half of the states in the US are keeping cancer patients from a potential life-saver or at the very least, life-improver, and causing some patients to commit illegal activities just to receive relief. Unfortunately, it isn't often economically viable for a person to relocate to an entire state just to receive their doctor's recommendation, and many are patiently waiting until their state decides to move towards legalization of medical marijuana.

Conclusion

You should now have a good understanding of medical marijuana, its history, laws, and be able to form an intelligent opinion on its use.

As you can see, there is still much more research needed to be done when it comes to medical marijuana. However, there is much evidence to show its benefits on anxiety, cancer, epilepsy, and more. As the drug becomes more accepted, there will be more studies done and progress being made to understand all its effects.

Made in the USA
San Bernardino, CA
11 March 2018